BREATH BEYOND LIMITS:

Overcoming Asthma Obstacles

DR. MELISSA P. NELSON

TABLE OF CONTENT

PREFACE

Welcome to "Breath Beyond Limits: Overcoming Asthma Obstacles." Asthma is a condition that affects millions of people worldwide, presenting unique challenges and obstacles that can sometimes feel insurmountable. Yet, within these challenges lie opportunities for growth, resilience, and empowerment.

As the author of this book, I have a deeply personal connection to asthma. Like many others, I have experienced firsthand the struggles of living with this condition – the breathlessness, the fear of attacks, and the limitations it can impose on daily life. However, I have also experienced the power of resilience and the ability to overcome obstacles with the right mindset, knowledge, and support.

The inspiration behind "Breath Beyond Limits" stems from my own journey with asthma and the desire to help others facing similar challenges. This book is not just about managing symptoms or avoiding triggers; it's about reclaiming control of your life and embracing the possibilities that lie beyond the limitations of asthma.

Throughout the pages of this book, you'll find practical strategies, insightful advice, and inspiring stories to guide you on your journey to overcoming asthma obstacles. From understanding your diagnosis and managing medications to staying active and navigating emotional challenges, each chapter is designed to empower you with the tools and knowledge you need to thrive with asthma.

Whether you're newly diagnosed or have been living with asthma for years, "Breath Beyond Limits" is here to support you every step of the way. It's a testament to the resilience of the human spirit and the power we all possess to overcome adversity and live life to the fullest.

I invite you to embark on this journey with an open heart and a willingness to embrace the possibilities that lie ahead.

Together, let's break free from the limitations of asthma and discover the boundless potential that exists within each and every one of us.

Introduction: Understanding Asthma

Asthma is a chronic respiratory condition that affects millions of people worldwide, making it imperative to grasp its fundamentals to navigate its challenges effectively. In this introductory section, we delve into the core aspects of asthma, shedding light on its definition, prevalence, symptoms, triggers, and the significance of proactive management for overall health and well-being.

Defining Asthma and Its Prevalence:

Asthma is a respiratory disorder characterized by inflammation and narrowing of the airways, leading to difficulty breathing, coughing, wheezing, and chest tightness. While the exact cause of asthma remains elusive, it often involves a combination of genetic predispositions and environmental factors.

The prevalence of asthma has surged in recent decades, with millions of individuals, both young and old, grappling with its impact on their daily lives. Across the globe, asthma affects people of all ages, ethnicities, and socioeconomic backgrounds, presenting a significant public health concern.

Overview of Common Symptoms and Triggers:

Understanding the symptoms and triggers of asthma is crucial for effectively managing the condition. Common symptoms include shortness of breath, chest tightness, wheezing (a whistling sound during breathing), and coughing, particularly at night or early morning.

Triggers are stimuli that can exacerbate asthma symptoms, leading to flare-ups or attacks. These triggers vary among individuals but may include allergens such as pollen, dust mites, pet dander, respiratory infections, air pollution, tobacco smoke, cold air, exercise, and stress.

Importance of Managing Asthma for Overall Health and Well-being:

Effective asthma management is paramount for maintaining optimal health and enhancing overall well-being. By diligently controlling symptoms and minimizing the risk of exacerbations, individuals with asthma can lead active, fulfilling lives.

Proactive management strategies may include:

1. Regularly monitoring symptoms and peak flow measurements.
2. Adhering to prescribed medication regimens, including controller and rescue medications.
3. Identifying and avoiding asthma triggers whenever possible.
4. Developing an asthma action plan in collaboration with healthcare providers.
5. Leading a healthy lifestyle through regular exercise, balanced nutrition, adequate sleep, and stress management techniques.

By taking proactive steps to manage asthma, individuals can reduce the frequency and severity of symptoms, enhance lung function, and improve overall quality of life.

In conclusion, understanding asthma is the first step towards effectively navigating its challenges. By defining asthma, recognizing its prevalence, understanding common symptoms and triggers, and emphasizing the importance of proactive management, individuals can embark on a journey towards better asthma control and improved well-being.

Through education, awareness, and empowerment, we can breathe easier and overcome the obstacles posed by asthma.

CHAPTER 1: Diagnosis and Understanding: Navigating the Asthma Journey

In the initial stages of the asthma journey, individuals often find themselves navigating a maze of symptoms, uncertainty, and questions. This chapter focuses on the pivotal steps of recognizing symptoms, seeking diagnosis, and gaining a deeper understanding of asthma's underlying causes and mechanisms. Additionally, it emphasizes the crucial role of asthma education for both patients and caregivers in managing the condition effectively.

Recognizing symptoms and seeking diagnosis

Asthma, a chronic respiratory condition, presents a diverse array of symptoms that can vary in severity and frequency among individuals. Recognizing these symptoms and promptly seeking diagnosis are crucial steps towards effectively managing asthma and improving quality of life.

Common Symptoms of Asthma:

1. Coughing: Persistent or recurrent coughing, particularly at night or in the early morning, is a hallmark symptom of asthma. This cough may be dry or accompanied by mucus production.

2. Wheezing: Wheezing refers to a high-pitched whistling sound heard during breathing, typically occurring when air flows through narrowed airways. It is often more noticeable during exhalation but may occur during inhalation as well.

3. Shortness of Breath: Asthma can cause a sensation of breathlessness or difficulty breathing, especially during physical exertion or exposure to triggers such as allergens or irritants. This shortness of breath may be mild or severe and may worsen over time if left untreated.

4. Chest Tightness: Individuals with asthma may experience a feeling of tightness or discomfort in the chest, often described as a pressure or squeezing sensation. This symptom can range from mild to severe and may occur intermittently or persistently.

5. Difficulty Breathing: Asthma can lead to a sensation of airway obstruction, making it challenging to inhale or exhale fully. This difficulty breathing may be accompanied by audible sounds such as wheezing or rattling in the chest.

Seeking Diagnosis:

When experiencing symptoms suggestive of asthma, it is essential to seek medical evaluation promptly. Diagnosis typically involves a comprehensive assessment by a healthcare professional, which may include the following steps:

1. Medical History: The healthcare provider will inquire about the individual's symptoms, medical history, family history of asthma or other respiratory conditions, and any potential triggers or exacerbating factors.

2. Physical Examination: A thorough physical examination, including lung auscultation (listening to breath sounds) and assessment of respiratory function, may be conducted to evaluate for signs of asthma.

3. Diagnostic Tests: Objective tests such as spirometry and peak flow measurement may be performed to assess lung function and airway responsiveness. These tests measure the amount and speed of air exhaled from the lungs, helping to diagnose and monitor asthma.

4. Allergy Testing: In some cases, allergy testing may be recommended to identify specific allergens that could trigger asthma symptoms. This may involve skin prick tests or blood tests to measure allergen-specific antibodies.

5. Other Investigations: Additional tests, such as chest X-rays or exhaled nitric oxide measurement, may be performed to rule out other respiratory conditions or assess airway inflammation.

By seeking timely diagnosis and collaborating with healthcare providers, individuals experiencing symptoms of asthma can initiate appropriate treatment and management strategies to improve asthma control and overall quality of life. Early intervention is key to preventing asthma exacerbations, reducing symptom severity, and minimizing long-term complications associated with uncontrolled asthma.

Understanding the underlying causes and mechanisms of asthma

Asthma is a complex respiratory condition characterized by inflammation and narrowing of the airways, leading to symptoms such as coughing, wheezing, shortness of breath, and chest tightness. While the exact causes of asthma remain incompletely understood, researchers have made significant strides in unraveling the underlying mechanisms that contribute to its development and progression.

Inflammation and Immune Dysregulation:

Central to the pathophysiology of asthma is airway inflammation, which involves an exaggerated immune response to various environmental triggers. In susceptible individuals, exposure to allergens, such as pollen, dust mites, pet dander, or air pollutants, can trigger an inflammatory cascade within the airways.

This inflammation is characterized by the recruitment and activation of immune cells, including eosinophils, mast cells, T lymphocytes, and macrophages. These immune cells release a variety of pro-inflammatory mediators, such as histamine, leukotrienes, and cytokines, which promote airway hyperresponsiveness and mucous production, leading to symptoms of asthma.

Airway Hyperresponsiveness:

Individuals with asthma often exhibit increased sensitivity and hyperreactivity of the airways to various stimuli. This heightened airway responsiveness predisposes them to exaggerated bronchoconstriction and airflow limitation in response to triggers such as allergens, respiratory infections, exercise, cold air, or irritants.

Airway Remodeling:

Chronic inflammation and repeated episodes of airway constriction in asthma can lead to structural changes in the airway walls, a process known as airway remodeling. These structural alterations include thickening of the airway smooth muscle, increased deposition of collagen and extracellular matrix proteins, and hypertrophy/hyperplasia of airway epithelial cells.

Airway remodeling contributes to persistent airflow limitation, reduced lung function, and increased susceptibility to asthma exacerbations. It represents a key feature of severe, persistent asthma and underscores the importance of early intervention to prevent irreversible changes in the airways.

Genetic and Environmental Factors:

While genetic predispositions play a role in asthma susceptibility, environmental exposures and gene-environment interactions also play significant roles in asthma development. Certain genetic variations related to immune function, airway epithelial integrity, and response to environmental triggers have been implicated in asthma susceptibility.

Environmental factors, including allergens, tobacco smoke, air pollution, respiratory infections, and socioeconomic disparities, can modulate gene expression and immune responses, contributing to asthma onset and exacerbations.

Understanding the complex interplay between genetic, environmental, and immune factors is crucial for developing targeted therapies and personalized treatment approaches for asthma. By targeting specific pathways involved in airway inflammation, hyperresponsiveness, and remodeling, researchers aim to improve asthma control, reduce exacerbations, and mitigate long-term complications associated with the condition.

In summary, asthma is a multifactorial respiratory condition characterized by airway inflammation, hyperresponsiveness, and remodeling. Genetic predispositions, environmental exposures, and immune dysregulation contribute to its development and progression. A deeper understanding of the underlying causes and mechanisms of asthma is essential for advancing research, developing effective treatments, and improving outcomes for individuals living with this chronic condition.

Importance of asthma education for patients and caregivers

Asthma education plays a pivotal role in empowering both patients and caregivers with the knowledge, skills, and confidence to effectively manage asthma and optimize outcomes. By providing comprehensive education, healthcare providers can empower individuals to take an active role in their asthma care, improve adherence to treatment regimens, and reduce the burden of asthma-related complications. Here are several key reasons why asthma education is essential:

1. Understanding the Condition: Asthma education provides individuals with a thorough understanding of asthma, including its causes, symptoms, triggers, and underlying mechanisms. By understanding the nature of their condition, patients and caregivers are better equipped to recognize symptoms, anticipate exacerbations, and respond promptly to changes in asthma control.

2. Medication Management: Proper use of asthma medications is essential for achieving and maintaining asthma control. Asthma education helps patients and caregivers understand the different types of asthma medications, their mechanisms of action, dosing schedules, and potential side effects. Education also emphasizes the importance of adherence to prescribed medication regimens and proper inhaler technique to ensure optimal medication delivery to the lungs.

3. Asthma Action Plans: Asthma action plans are personalized documents developed in collaboration with healthcare providers that outline steps to take in response to changes in asthma symptoms or peak flow measurements.

These plans typically include instructions for adjusting medication dosages, recognizing early warning signs of worsening asthma, and seeking medical attention when necessary. Asthma education ensures that patients and caregivers understand their asthma action plan and feel confident in implementing it during asthma exacerbations.

4. Identifying and Avoiding Triggers: Asthma education helps individuals identify common asthma triggers, such as allergens, irritants, respiratory infections, and exercise, and learn strategies to minimize exposure to these triggers. By avoiding triggers whenever possible and implementing preventive measures, patients can reduce the frequency and severity of asthma symptoms and exacerbations.

5. Lifestyle Modifications: Asthma education emphasizes the importance of lifestyle modifications in managing asthma effectively. This may include maintaining a healthy weight, engaging in regular physical activity, avoiding tobacco smoke and other respiratory irritants, and managing stress. By adopting a healthy lifestyle, individuals can improve lung function, enhance overall well-being, and reduce the risk of asthma exacerbations.

6. Communication with Healthcare Providers: Effective communication between patients and healthcare providers is essential for optimizing asthma management. Asthma education encourages open dialogue between patients, caregivers, and healthcare providers, fostering collaborative decision-making and ensuring that treatment plans align with individual needs and preferences.

7. Empowerment and Self-Advocacy: Asthma education empowers patients and caregivers to become active participants in their asthma care, advocating for their health needs and making informed decisions about their treatment. By providing individuals with the knowledge and skills to manage their asthma effectively, education promotes self-efficacy and confidence in managing the condition.

In conclusion, asthma education is a cornerstone of effective asthma management, empowering patients and caregivers with the knowledge, skills, and confidence to navigate the complexities of asthma and achieve optimal outcomes. By understanding the condition, adhering to medication regimens, implementing asthma action plans, identifying and avoiding triggers, adopting healthy lifestyle behaviors, communicating with healthcare providers, and advocating for their health needs, individuals can take control of their asthma and lead fulfilling lives.

CHAPTER 2: Medication Management: Finding the Right Treatment Approach

Medication management is a cornerstone of effective asthma care, aiming to control symptoms, prevent exacerbations, and improve overall quality of life. This chapter provides an overview of asthma medications, their roles in asthma management, understanding inhalers, nebulizers, and other delivery devices, and strategies for adherence to medication regimens.

Overview of Asthma Medications and Their Roles

Asthma is a chronic respiratory condition characterized by inflammation and narrowing of the airways, leading to symptoms such as coughing, wheezing, shortness of breath, and chest tightness. Effective management of asthma typically involves the use of various medications aimed at controlling symptoms, reducing airway inflammation, preventing exacerbations, and improving overall lung function.

Here is an overview of the main classes of asthma medications and their roles in asthma management:

1. Inhaled Corticosteroids (ICS):

- **Role:** ICS medications are the cornerstone of asthma therapy and work by reducing airway inflammation, thereby preventing asthma symptoms and exacerbations.

- **Mechanism of Action:** ICS medications exert their anti-inflammatory effects by suppressing the production of inflammatory mediators and inhibiting the recruitment and activation of inflammatory cells in the airways.

- **Examples:** Beclomethasone, Budesonide, Fluticasone, Mometasone.

2. Long-Acting Beta-Agonists (LABAs):

- **Role:** LABAs are bronchodilators that help relax and widen the airways, providing long-term symptom control when used in combination with ICS medications.

- **Mechanism of Action:** LABAs stimulate beta-adrenergic receptors in the airway smooth muscle, leading to bronchodilation and improved airflow.

- **Examples:** Formoterol, Salmeterol, Vilanterol.

3. Leukotriene Modifiers:

- **Role:** Leukotriene modifiers block the action of leukotrienes, inflammatory substances that contribute to airway inflammation and constriction, thereby reducing asthma symptoms and improving lung function.

- **Mechanism of Action:** Leukotriene modifiers inhibit the production or activity of leukotrienes, which play a key role in the inflammatory cascade in asthma.

- **Examples:** Montelukast, Zafirlukast, Zileuton.

4. Immunomodulators:

- **Role:** Immunomodulators are biologic medications that target specific immune pathways involved in asthma inflammation, providing targeted therapy for severe, uncontrolled asthma.

- **Mechanism of Action:** Immunomodulators interfere with immune mediators, such as immunoglobulin E (IgE) or interleukin-5 (IL-5), to reduce airway inflammation and prevent asthma exacerbations.

- **Examples:** Omalizumab (anti-IgE), Mepolizumab, Reslizumab, Benralizumab (anti-IL-5).

5. Short-Acting Beta-Agonists (SABAs):

- **Role:** SABAs are rescue medications used for quick relief of acute asthma symptoms and bronchoconstriction during asthma attacks or exacerbations.

- **Mechanism of Action:** SABAs stimulate beta-adrenergic receptors in the airway smooth muscle, leading to rapid bronchodilation and improved airflow.

- **Examples:** Albuterol (salbutamol), Levalbuterol, Terbutaline.

6. Oral Corticosteroids:

- **Role:** Oral corticosteroids are used to treat severe asthma exacerbations or persistent asthma symptoms that are not controlled with other medications.

- **Mechanism of Action:** Oral corticosteroids exert potent anti-inflammatory effects throughout the body, suppressing the immune response and reducing airway inflammation.

- **Examples:** Prednisone, Prednisolone, Methylprednisolone.

Individuals with asthma may require a combination of these medications, tailored to their specific needs and asthma severity. It is essential for healthcare providers to carefully assess asthma control, adjust treatment regimens as needed, and monitor for medication side effects to ensure optimal asthma management and improve overall quality of life.

Understanding Inhalers, Nebulizers, and Other Delivery Devices

Inhalers, nebulizers, and other delivery devices are essential tools for administering asthma medications directly to the lungs, where they can effectively relieve symptoms, reduce airway inflammation, and improve lung function. Understanding how these devices work and how to use them correctly is crucial for achieving optimal asthma management. Here's an overview of the main types of inhalers, nebulizers, and other delivery devices used in asthma treatment:

1. Metered-Dose Inhalers (MDIs):

- **Description:** Metered-dose inhalers deliver a measured dose of medication in aerosol form, which is inhaled into the lungs.

- **Mechanism of Action:** With each inhalation, the device releases a predetermined amount of medication, which is propelled into the airways.

- **How to Use:** Shake the inhaler before each use, exhale fully, place the mouthpiece between the lips, and inhale deeply and slowly while simultaneously pressing down on the canister to release the medication. Hold the breath for a few seconds before exhaling slowly.

- **Examples:** Albuterol (salbutamol) MDI, Fluticasone MDI, Budesonide/Formoterol combination MDI.

2. Dry Powder Inhalers (DPIs):

- **Description:** Dry powder inhalers deliver medication in powder form, which is inhaled into the lungs when activated by the patient's inhalation.

- **Mechanism of Action:** DPIs rely on the patient's inspiratory effort to disperse the medication powder into the airways.

- **How to Use:** Load the medication dose into the inhaler device, exhale fully, place the mouthpiece between the lips, and inhale forcefully and deeply to disperse the powder into the lungs. Hold the breath for a few seconds before exhaling slowly.

- **Examples:** Fluticasone/Salmeterol DPI, Formoterol DPI, Budesonide DPI.

3. Soft Mist Inhalers (SMIs):

- **Description:** Soft mist inhalers deliver medication in a fine mist form, which is inhaled into the lungs through a slow and steady inhalation.

- **Mechanism of Action:** SMIs produce a soft mist of medication using a propellant system, allowing for slower inhalation compared to MDIs.

  - **How to Use:** Prime the inhaler before first use, exhale fully, place the mouthpiece between the lips, and inhale slowly and deeply to inhale the mist. Hold the breath for a few seconds before exhaling slowly.

  - **Examples:** Respimat inhaler (Tiotropium Bromide), Combivent Respimat (Ipratropium/Albuterol).

4. Nebulizers:

  - **Description:** Nebulizers convert liquid medication into a fine mist that can be inhaled through a mask or mouthpiece.

  - **Mechanism of Action:** Nebulizers use compressed air or ultrasonic vibrations to aerosolize the medication solution, delivering it directly into the airways.

  - **How to Use:** Place the medication solution into the nebulizer chamber, attach the mask or mouthpiece, and inhale the mist generated by the nebulizer for the prescribed duration.

  - **Examples:** Jet nebulizers, ultrasonic nebulizers, mesh nebulizers.

In addition to these primary inhalation devices, other delivery devices such as spacer devices and valved holding chambers (VHCs) are often used with MDIs to improve medication delivery and reduce the risk of oral deposition.

These devices help coordinate the timing of medication release with inhalation, ensuring optimal drug delivery to the lungs.

Proper technique and adherence to medication regimens are essential for maximizing the effectiveness of inhalers, nebulizers, and other delivery devices in asthma management. Healthcare providers should provide thorough education and training on device use, monitor inhaler technique regularly, and address any barriers to adherence to ensure optimal asthma control and improve patient outcomes.

Strategies for Adherence to Medication Regimens

Adherence to prescribed medication regimens is critical for achieving and maintaining optimal asthma control, reducing the risk of exacerbations, and improving overall quality of life for individuals with asthma. However, adherence to medication regimens can be challenging for various reasons, including forgetfulness, concerns about side effects, difficulty using inhaler devices, and misconceptions about the necessity of medication. Implementing strategies to promote adherence is essential for optimizing asthma management. Here are several effective strategies for improving adherence to medication regimens in asthma:

1. Education and Counseling: Provide comprehensive education about asthma medications, their roles in managing asthma, and the importance of adherence to treatment regimens. Address any concerns or misconceptions about medications and clarify the benefits of long-term asthma control.

2. Simplify Regimens: Simplify medication regimens by reducing the number of medications whenever possible and using combination inhalers that contain multiple medications in a single device. Once-daily dosing options may also improve convenience and adherence.

3. Use of Reminder Systems: Implement reminder systems to help patients remember to take their medications regularly. This may include medication calendars, pill organizers, smartphone apps, or alarms. Encourage patients to incorporate medication doses into their daily routines, such as taking medications with meals or at bedtime.

4. Regular Follow-Up: Schedule regular follow-up appointments with healthcare providers to monitor asthma control, assess medication adherence, and adjust treatment regimens as needed. Use these opportunities to address any barriers to adherence and provide additional education and support.

5. Visual Aids and Written Instructions: Provide visual aids, written instructions, or demonstration videos to reinforce proper inhaler technique and ensure that patients understand how to use their inhaler devices correctly. Encourage patients to demonstrate their inhaler technique during clinic visits to identify and correct any errors.

6. Tailored Approach: Take a personalized approach to asthma management by considering individual patient preferences, lifestyle factors, and socioeconomic barriers to adherence. Involve patients in shared decision-making regarding their treatment plan and address any concerns or preferences regarding medication options.

7. Family and Caregiver Support: Involve family members or caregivers in the asthma management process and educate them about the importance of medication adherence. Encourage open communication and collaboration among family members to provide support and reinforcement for medication adherence.

8. Addressing Barriers and Concerns: Take the time to listen to patients' concerns and address any barriers to adherence they may be experiencing. This may include addressing concerns about medication side effects, cost, or difficulty using inhaler devices. Provide reassurance, support, and solutions to address these barriers.

9. Patient Engagement and Empowerment: Empower patients to take an active role in their asthma management and decision-making regarding their treatment. Encourage self-monitoring of symptoms, adherence to treatment regimens, and communication with healthcare providers about any changes in asthma control.

10. Positive Reinforcement: Provide positive reinforcement and recognition for patients who demonstrate good adherence to their medication regimens. Celebrate milestones and achievements in asthma control and emphasize the benefits of adherence to long-term health outcomes.

By implementing these strategies, healthcare providers can help individuals with asthma overcome barriers to adherence and improve their ability to manage their condition effectively. Promoting adherence to medication regimens is essential for optimizing asthma control, reducing the risk of exacerbations, and improving overall quality of life for individuals living with asthma.

CHAPTER 3: Lifestyle Modifications: Creating an Asthma-Friendly Environment

Living with asthma requires a proactive approach to managing triggers, maintaining asthma control, and improving overall well-being. This chapter focuses on lifestyle modifications aimed at creating an asthma-friendly environment, both at home and in the workplace. It covers strategies for identifying and minimizing asthma triggers, creating an asthma action plan for daily management, and incorporating asthma-friendly habits into daily life.

Identifying and Minimizing Asthma Triggers in the Home and Workplace

Asthma triggers are substances or environmental factors that can exacerbate asthma symptoms or lead to asthma attacks in susceptible individuals. Identifying and minimizing these triggers is essential for effectively managing asthma and reducing the frequency and severity of symptoms. Here are some strategies for identifying and minimizing asthma triggers in both the home and workplace:

- **Home Environment:**

1. Allergens:

- **Dust Mites:** Use allergen-proof mattress and pillow covers, wash bedding weekly in hot water (130°F or higher), and vacuum carpets and upholstery regularly using a vacuum cleaner with a high-efficiency particulate air (HEPA) filter.

- **Pet Dander:** If you have pets, keep them out of the bedroom, bathe them regularly, and vacuum upholstered furniture and carpets frequently.

- **Mold:** Keep indoor humidity levels below 50% by using a dehumidifier, fixing leaks promptly, and regularly cleaning damp areas such as bathrooms and basements.

2. Tobacco Smoke:

- Avoid smoking indoors and discourage guests from smoking inside the home. Consider implementing a smoke-free policy in the household to protect individuals with asthma from secondhand smoke exposure.

3. Airborne Irritants:

- Use exhaust fans or open windows when cooking to reduce exposure to cooking fumes and odors.

- Minimize the use of strong-smelling cleaning products, air fresheners, and scented candles, as these can trigger asthma symptoms in some individuals.

- Keep indoor air clean by using HEPA air purifiers and regularly changing air filters in heating and cooling systems.

- **Workplace Environment:**

1. Occupational Exposures:

- Identify potential asthma triggers in the workplace, such as dust, chemicals, fumes, or allergens specific to certain occupations.

- Work with employers to implement measures to reduce exposure to workplace triggers, such as improving ventilation, using personal protective equipment (e.g., masks or respirators), and substituting hazardous substances with safer alternatives.

- Follow recommended safety protocols and training procedures to minimize the risk of occupational asthma, especially in high-risk industries such as manufacturing, construction, healthcare, and agriculture.

2. Secondhand Smoke:

- Advocate for smoke-free policies in the workplace to protect individuals with asthma from exposure to secondhand smoke.

- Designate smoking areas away from entrances and ventilation intakes to prevent smoke from infiltrating indoor spaces.

3. Environmental Controls:

- Implement engineering controls, such as local exhaust ventilation systems or enclosures, to minimize exposure to airborne contaminants and pollutants in the workplace.

- Provide adequate ventilation in indoor spaces by ensuring proper airflow and air exchange rates, especially in areas where chemical or fume exposure is a concern.

4. Education and Awareness:

- Educate employees and employers about the potential health effects of workplace exposures on asthma and the importance of implementing preventive measures to create a safe and healthy work environment.

- Encourage regular communication between workers and management regarding any concerns or observations related to workplace hazards or asthma triggers.

By identifying and minimizing asthma triggers in both the home and workplace, individuals with asthma can reduce the likelihood of asthma symptoms and exacerbations, improve asthma control, and enhance overall quality of life. Working collaboratively with healthcare providers, employers, and other stakeholders is essential for implementing effective strategies to create asthma-friendly environments and support the well-being of individuals living with asthma.

Creating an Asthma Action Plan for Daily Management

An asthma action plan is a personalized document developed in collaboration with healthcare providers that outlines steps to take for managing asthma on a day-to-day basis. It provides clear instructions for adjusting medication dosages, recognizing early warning signs of worsening asthma, and seeking medical attention when necessary. An asthma action plan empowers individuals with asthma and their caregivers to take an active role in managing the condition effectively.

Here are the key components of an asthma action plan:

- **Personal Information:**
  - The asthma action plan should include basic personal information, including the individual's name, date of birth, emergency contact information, and healthcare provider's contact details.

- **Asthma Severity Classification:**
  - Asthma action plans typically classify asthma severity into categories such as intermittent, mild persistent, moderate persistent, or severe persistent, based on symptom frequency, nighttime awakenings, and lung function measurements.

- **Medication Management:**
  - The action plan should include a list of prescribed asthma medications, including controller medications (e.g., inhaled corticosteroids, long-acting beta-agonists) for daily maintenance and rescue medications (e.g., short-acting beta-agonists) for quick relief of symptoms.
  - Specific instructions should be provided for each medication, including dosages, frequency of use, and proper inhaler technique.

- **Peak Flow Monitoring:**

- If peak flow monitoring is part of the asthma management plan, the action plan should include instructions for measuring peak flow using a peak flow meter, interpreting peak flow readings, and determining appropriate actions based on peak flow measurements.

- **Asthma Zones:**
- Asthma action plans typically divide asthma symptoms into color-coded zones to indicate the level of asthma control and corresponding actions to take:

- **Green Zone (Good Control):** Indicates stable asthma with no symptoms or minimal symptoms. Instructions may include continuing regular medication use and monitoring symptoms.

- **Yellow Zone (Caution):** Indicates worsening asthma with increased symptoms or decreased peak flow readings. Instructions may include stepping up controller medication use and monitoring symptoms more closely.

- **Red Zone (Medical Alert):** Indicates severe asthma exacerbation requiring immediate medical attention. Instructions may include using rescue medications, seeking emergency medical care, and contacting healthcare providers.

- **Symptom Recognition and Response:**

- The action plan should provide clear guidance on recognizing early warning signs of worsening asthma, such as increased coughing, wheezing, shortness of breath, chest tightness, or changes in peak flow readings.
- Specific actions to take in response to worsening symptoms should be outlined for each asthma zone, including adjustments to medication dosages, initiating rescue medication use, and seeking medical evaluation.

- **Emergency Contact Information:**
- The action plan should include emergency contact information for healthcare providers, including phone numbers for primary care physicians, asthma specialists, and emergency medical services.

- **Follow-Up and Review:**
- The action plan should specify when to schedule follow-up appointments with healthcare providers for asthma management review and adjustment of treatment plans as needed.

Asthma action plans should be tailored to individual needs, asthma severity, and treatment preferences. They should be reviewed and updated regularly in collaboration with healthcare providers to ensure that they reflect current asthma control and provide effective guidance for daily asthma management. By following an asthma action plan, individuals with asthma can take proactive steps to monitor symptoms, adjust medication use, and seek appropriate medical care, leading to better asthma control and improved quality of life.

Tips for Incorporating Asthma-Friendly Habits into Daily Life

Living with asthma requires proactive management and lifestyle adjustments to minimize triggers, maintain asthma control, and improve overall well-being. Incorporating asthma-friendly habits into daily life can help individuals with asthma manage their condition more effectively and reduce the frequency and severity of symptoms.
Here are some practical tips for integrating asthma-friendly habits into daily routines:

1. Regular Medication Adherence:
- Take prescribed asthma medications as directed by healthcare providers, including controller medications for long-term maintenance and rescue medications for quick relief of symptoms.

- Set reminders or alarms to ensure timely medication doses and establish a routine for medication administration.

2. Environmental Awareness:

- Stay informed about potential asthma triggers in the environment, such as pollen, air pollution, cold air, dust mites, pet dander, mold, and smoke.

- Check air quality forecasts and pollen counts regularly, especially during allergy seasons, and limit outdoor activities on days with high pollution or pollen levels.

3. Indoor Air Quality:

- Maintain good indoor air quality by keeping indoor spaces clean, well-ventilated, and free of dust, mold, and other allergens.

- Use high-efficiency particulate air (HEPA) filters in vacuum cleaners and air purifiers to remove airborne allergens and pollutants.

4. Allergen Control:

- Implement allergen control measures in the home, such as using allergen-proof mattress and pillow covers, washing bedding in hot water weekly, and vacuuming carpets and upholstery regularly.

- Minimize exposure to pet dander by keeping pets out of the bedroom, bathing them regularly, and vacuuming upholstered furniture and carpets frequently.

5. Smoke-Free Environment:

- Avoid exposure to tobacco smoke and secondhand smoke, as it can trigger asthma symptoms and exacerbate respiratory problems.

- Advocate for smoke-free policies in the home, workplace, and public spaces to protect individuals with asthma from the harmful effects of smoking.

6. Regular Exercise:

- Engage in regular physical activity and exercise to improve lung function, cardiovascular health, and overall fitness.

- Choose asthma-friendly activities such as swimming, walking, cycling, or yoga, and warm up before exercise to reduce the risk of exercise-induced asthma symptoms.

7. Stress Management:

- Practice stress-reduction techniques such as deep breathing exercises, meditation, mindfulness, or relaxation techniques to manage stress and anxiety, which can exacerbate asthma symptoms.

- Prioritize self-care activities, hobbies, and leisure activities that promote relaxation and well-being.

8. Healthy Lifestyle Choices:

- Maintain a healthy diet rich in fruits, vegetables, whole grains, and lean proteins to support overall health and immune function.
- Stay hydrated by drinking plenty of water throughout the day, as dehydration can worsen asthma symptoms.

9. Asthma Education and Self-Management:

- Stay educated about asthma management strategies, medication use, inhaler techniques, and asthma action plans.
- Keep track of asthma symptoms, peak flow measurements, and triggers in a diary or journal to identify patterns and trends over time.

10. Regular Healthcare Follow-Up:

- Schedule regular follow-up appointments with healthcare providers for asthma management review, monitoring of lung function, and adjustment of treatment plans as needed.
- Communicate openly with healthcare providers about any changes in asthma symptoms, medication side effects, or concerns about asthma management.

By incorporating these asthma-friendly habits into daily life, individuals with asthma can better manage their condition, reduce the impact of triggers, and improve overall asthma control and quality of life. Consistency, awareness, and proactive self-care are key to successfully managing asthma and minimizing the risk of asthma exacerbations.

CHAPTER 4: Exercise and Physical Activity: Overcoming Challenges and Staying Active

Regular exercise and physical activity play a crucial role in asthma management, contributing to improved lung function, cardiovascular health, and overall well-being. However, individuals with asthma may face unique challenges when participating in physical activity, including concerns about triggering asthma symptoms or exacerbations. This chapter explores the importance of exercise for asthma management, strategies for safely participating in physical activity with asthma, and tips for managing exercise-induced symptoms and staying motivated.

Importance of Exercise for Asthma Management

Exercise is a crucial component of asthma management, offering numerous benefits for individuals with asthma in terms of both physical and psychological health. Despite concerns about triggering asthma symptoms, regular physical activity can significantly improve asthma control and overall well-being. Here are some key reasons why exercise is important for asthma management:

1. Improved Lung Function: Regular exercise helps strengthen the respiratory muscles and improve lung function. It promotes deeper breathing, enhances ventilation, and increases lung capacity, leading to better oxygen exchange and respiratory efficiency. Stronger lungs are better equipped to handle the challenges posed by asthma, reducing the severity and frequency of symptoms.

2. Enhanced Cardiovascular Fitness: Engaging in aerobic exercise improves cardiovascular fitness and endurance, enhancing heart and lung function. Cardiovascular exercise strengthens the heart muscle, improves circulation, and increases oxygen delivery to tissues, contributing to overall cardiovascular health. Improved cardiovascular fitness enables individuals with asthma to tolerate physical exertion more effectively and reduces the risk of fatigue and breathlessness during activities of daily living.

3. Weight Management: Regular physical activity plays a key role in weight management and obesity prevention. Maintaining a healthy weight is essential for individuals with asthma, as obesity is associated with increased asthma severity, poorer asthma control, and higher rates of asthma-related hospitalizations. Exercise helps regulate metabolism, burn calories, and promote weight loss, thereby reducing the burden on the respiratory system and improving asthma control.

4. Reduced Inflammation: Exercise has anti-inflammatory effects on the body, reducing systemic inflammation and modulating immune responses. In individuals with asthma, regular exercise can help mitigate airway inflammation and hyperresponsiveness, leading to fewer asthma symptoms and reduced reliance on medication. Exercise-induced anti-inflammatory effects may contribute to improved asthma control and reduced risk of exacerbations.

5. Psychological Benefits: Exercise has numerous psychological benefits, including stress reduction, mood enhancement, and anxiety relief. Physical activity stimulates the release of endorphins, neurotransmitters that promote feelings of happiness and well-being. Regular exercise can help alleviate symptoms of depression and anxiety, which are common comorbidities in individuals with asthma. By promoting mental health and emotional resilience, exercise contributes to overall quality of life and coping with the challenges of living with asthma.

Despite the potential benefits of exercise for asthma management, individuals with asthma may face barriers to physical activity, such as fear of triggering asthma symptoms, lack of confidence, or misconceptions about exercise-induced bronchoconstriction. However, with proper guidance, monitoring, and self-care, individuals with asthma can safely participate in a variety of physical activities and reap the many rewards of an active lifestyle. Incorporating exercise into asthma management plans can lead to improved asthma control, enhanced physical fitness, and better overall health outcomes.

Strategies for Safely Participating in Physical Activity with Asthma

Regular physical activity is important for overall health and well-being, including for individuals with asthma. However, concerns about triggering asthma symptoms during exercise may deter some individuals from being physically active. With proper planning and precautions, individuals with asthma can safely participate in a wide range of activities. Here are some strategies for safely engaging in physical activity with asthma:

1. Consult Healthcare Provider:

- Before starting an exercise program, consult with a healthcare provider, such as a primary care physician or asthma specialist. They can assess asthma control, provide personalized recommendations, and suggest appropriate exercise regimens based on individual needs and asthma severity.

2. Warm-Up and Cool Down:

- Always start with a gentle warm-up before exercise to prepare the body for physical activity. A warm-up session of 5 to 10 minutes of light aerobic exercise, such as walking or cycling, can help gradually increase heart rate and respiratory rate. Similarly, end each exercise session with a cool-down period to gradually decrease heart rate and respiratory rate. Cooling down can include stretching exercises to improve flexibility and reduce muscle soreness.

3. Choose Asthma-Friendly Activities:

- Opt for activities that are less likely to trigger asthma symptoms. Swimming, walking, cycling, yoga, and tai chi are generally well-tolerated by individuals with asthma because they involve steady, rhythmic breathing and are performed in warm, humid environments. Avoid activities that involve prolonged exposure to cold, dry air, such as ice hockey or cross-country skiing, as cold air can trigger bronchoconstriction in some individuals with asthma.

4. Use Bronchodilator Before Exercise:

- Take a short-acting bronchodilator, such as albuterol, before exercise to open up the airways and prevent exercise-induced bronchoconstriction (EIB). Bronchodilators can be administered via inhaler or nebulizer approximately 15 to 30 minutes before exercise. Always follow healthcare provider's instructions regarding medication use.

5. Monitor Symptoms:

- Pay close attention to asthma symptoms during exercise and adjust the intensity or duration of activity accordingly. Common signs of exercise-induced bronchoconstriction include coughing, wheezing, chest tightness, and shortness of breath. If symptoms occur, take a break, use a rescue inhaler if needed, and wait until symptoms subside before resuming activity.

6. Stay Hydrated:

- Drink plenty of fluids before, during, and after exercise to stay hydrated. Dehydration can worsen asthma symptoms and increase the risk of bronchoconstriction. Water is the best choice for hydration, but sports drinks may be beneficial for prolonged or intense exercise sessions to replenish electrolytes lost through sweating.

7. Avoid Outdoor Allergens:

- If outdoor allergens trigger asthma symptoms, schedule outdoor activities when pollen levels are low, such as early morning or late evening. Check local pollen forecasts and air quality reports before exercising outdoors, and consider wearing a mask or scarf to cover the nose and mouth to reduce inhalation of allergens.

8. Listen to Your Body:

- Listen to your body and know your limits. It's important to recognize when to push through discomfort and when to take a break. Avoid overexertion and gradual increase the intensity and duration of exercise over time to build endurance safely.

9. Carry Rescue Medication:

- Always carry a rescue inhaler with you during exercise in case of an asthma flare-up. Know how to use it properly and have a plan in place for seeking medical help if needed.

By following these strategies, individuals with asthma can safely participate in physical activity, enjoy the numerous health benefits of exercise, and improve asthma control and overall quality of life. Consistency, caution, and proper preparation are key to successful and enjoyable physical activity with asthma.

Tips for Managing Exercise-Induced Symptoms and Staying Motivated

Exercise-induced symptoms can be challenging for individuals with asthma, but with proper management strategies and motivation, it's possible to overcome these obstacles and enjoy the benefits of physical activity. Here are some tips for managing exercise-induced symptoms and staying motivated:

1. Know Your Triggers:
- Identify specific triggers that may exacerbate asthma symptoms during exercise, such as cold air, pollen, air pollution, or allergens. Avoiding or minimizing exposure to these triggers can help reduce the risk of symptoms.

2. Use Medication Prophylactically:

- Take prescribed asthma medications, such as bronchodilators or controller medications, as recommended by your healthcare provider, before exercise. Using medication prophylactically can help prevent exercise-induced bronchoconstriction and improve exercise tolerance.

3. Warm-Up Adequately:

- Always start with a thorough warm-up before engaging in strenuous exercise. A warm-up helps prepare the body for physical activity by gradually increasing heart rate, blood flow, and respiratory rate. Incorporate dynamic stretches and gentle movements to loosen muscles and joints.

4. Practice Proper Breathing Techniques:

- Focus on proper breathing techniques during exercise to optimize oxygen intake and reduce the risk of hyperventilation or breathlessness. Practice diaphragmatic breathing, inhaling deeply through the nose and exhaling slowly through the mouth.

5. Monitor Symptoms Closely:

- Pay close attention to asthma symptoms during exercise, such as coughing, wheezing, chest tightness, or shortness of breath. If symptoms occur, take a break, use a rescue inhaler if needed, and wait until symptoms subside before resuming activity.

6. Choose Asthma-Friendly Activities:

- Opt for activities that are less likely to trigger asthma symptoms, such as swimming, walking, cycling, or yoga. These activities involve steady, rhythmic breathing and are performed in warm, humid environments, making them more asthma-friendly.

7. Stay Hydrated:

- Drink plenty of fluids before, during, and after exercise to stay hydrated. Dehydration can worsen asthma symptoms, so it's essential to replenish fluids regularly. Water is the best choice for hydration, but sports drinks may be beneficial for prolonged or intense exercise sessions.

8. Cool Down Properly:

- End each exercise session with a cool-down period to gradually decrease heart rate and respiratory rate. Incorporate static stretches to improve flexibility and reduce muscle tension. Cooling down helps prevent post-exercise symptoms and promotes recovery.

9. Listen to Your Body:

- Listen to your body and know your limits. Don't push yourself too hard, especially if you're experiencing asthma symptoms or fatigue. It's important to recognize when to take a break and when to continue exercising.

10. Stay Motivated:

- Set realistic goals for exercise and celebrate your achievements along the way. Find activities that you enjoy and incorporate variety into your exercise routine to keep things interesting. Consider exercising with a friend or joining a group fitness class for added motivation and accountability.

11. Track Your Progress:

- Keep a log of your exercise sessions, including the type of activity, duration, intensity, and any symptoms experienced. Tracking your progress can help you identify patterns, monitor improvements, and adjust your exercise routine as needed.

12. Seek Support:

- Don't hesitate to reach out to healthcare providers, fitness professionals, or support groups for guidance and encouragement. Surround yourself with a supportive network of friends, family, and peers who understand your challenges and can offer encouragement along your fitness journey.

By implementing these tips, individuals with asthma can effectively manage exercise-induced symptoms, stay motivated, and enjoy the many benefits of physical activity. With proper preparation, monitoring, and self-care, exercise can become a rewarding and enjoyable part of life with asthma.

CHAPTER 5: Nutrition and Diet: Fueling Your Body for Asthma Wellness

Nutrition and diet play a significant role in asthma management, influencing inflammation, immune function, and overall respiratory health. This chapter explores the importance of diet in asthma management, identifies asthma-friendly foods and nutrients, and provides tips for meal planning and navigating dietary restrictions.

Understanding the Role of Diet in Asthma Management

Diet plays a crucial role in asthma management, influencing inflammation, immune function, and overall respiratory health. While diet alone cannot cure asthma, adopting a nutritious eating plan can help individuals with asthma better manage their condition and reduce the frequency and severity of symptoms.

Here's an overview of how diet impacts asthma management:

1. Inflammation Control:

- Chronic inflammation is a hallmark feature of asthma, contributing to airway constriction, mucus production, and respiratory symptoms. Certain dietary factors can either promote or reduce inflammation in the body.

- An anti-inflammatory diet, characterized by the consumption of fruits, vegetables, whole grains, healthy fats, and lean proteins, may help mitigate inflammation and decrease the risk of asthma exacerbations.

- Foods rich in antioxidants, such as berries, leafy greens, nuts, seeds, and fatty fish, can help neutralize harmful free radicals and reduce oxidative stress, which contributes to inflammation in the airways.

2. Immune Function:

- A well-balanced diet supports immune function, helping the body defend against infections and allergens that can trigger asthma symptoms. Nutrient-rich foods provide essential vitamins, minerals, and antioxidants that support immune health and respiratory function.

- Adequate intake of vitamin C, vitamin D, zinc, selenium, and other immune-supporting nutrients may help strengthen the immune system and reduce susceptibility to respiratory infections and asthma exacerbations.

3. Weight Management:

- Maintaining a healthy weight is important for asthma management, as obesity is associated with increased asthma severity and reduced lung function. A balanced diet that includes appropriate portion sizes and emphasizes nutrient-dense foods can support weight management and improve asthma control.

- Consuming a diet high in fruits, vegetables, whole grains, and lean proteins while limiting processed foods, sugary beverages, and high-calorie snacks can help individuals maintain a healthy weight and reduce the risk of obesity-related asthma complications.

4. Gut Health:

- Emerging research suggests that the gut microbiome may play a role in asthma development and severity. A diet rich in fiber, prebiotics, and probiotics supports a diverse and balanced gut microbiota, which may help regulate immune responses and reduce inflammation in the airways.

- Fermented foods such as yogurt, kefir, sauerkraut, and kimchi contain beneficial probiotic bacteria that support gut health and may have positive effects on asthma symptoms.

5. Hydration:

- Proper hydration is essential for respiratory health and mucous membrane function. Drinking an adequate amount of water throughout the day helps keep airways moist and supports optimal lung function.

- Individuals with asthma should aim to drink plenty of fluids, primarily water, to stay hydrated. Avoiding excessive caffeine and alcohol consumption, which can have dehydrating effects, is also important for maintaining hydration levels.

By understanding the role of diet in asthma management and adopting a balanced eating plan that emphasizes nutrient-rich foods, individuals with asthma can better support their respiratory health, reduce inflammation, and improve asthma control. Working with a registered dietitian or healthcare provider can provide personalized nutrition guidance and support tailored to individual needs and dietary preferences.

Identifying Asthma-Friendly Foods and Nutrients

Choosing the right foods and nutrients can play a significant role in managing asthma symptoms and supporting overall respiratory health. While there is no specific "asthma diet," incorporating certain foods and nutrients into your meals may help reduce inflammation, support immune function, and improve asthma control. Here are some asthma-friendly foods and nutrients to include in your diet:

1. Antioxidant-Rich Foods:

- Antioxidants are compounds that help neutralize harmful free radicals and reduce oxidative stress in the body. By reducing inflammation, antioxidants can help alleviate asthma symptoms and improve lung function.

- Include a variety of colorful fruits and vegetables in your diet, such as berries (blueberries, strawberries, raspberries), citrus fruits (oranges, lemons, grapefruits), leafy greens (spinach, kale, Swiss chard), tomatoes, bell peppers, and sweet potatoes.

- Other antioxidant-rich foods include nuts (especially almonds and walnuts), seeds (flaxseeds, chia seeds), and herbs and spices (turmeric, ginger, cinnamon).

2. Omega-3 Fatty Acids:

- Omega-3 fatty acids are polyunsaturated fats with anti-inflammatory properties. They can help reduce airway inflammation and improve lung function in individuals with asthma.

- Incorporate fatty fish into your diet two to three times per week, such as salmon, mackerel, sardines, trout, and tuna. These fish are rich sources of eicosapentaenoic acid (EPA) and docosahexaenoic acid (DHA), two types of omega-3 fatty acids.

- Plant-based sources of omega-3 fatty acids include flaxseeds, chia seeds, hemp seeds, walnuts, and algae-derived supplements.

3. Vitamin D:

- Adequate vitamin D levels are important for immune function and respiratory health. Low vitamin D levels have been associated with increased asthma risk and severity.

- Get vitamin D from sunlight exposure and dietary sources such as fatty fish (salmon, mackerel, sardines), fortified dairy products (milk, yogurt, cheese), fortified plant-based milk alternatives, egg yolks, and mushrooms.

4. Magnesium:

- Magnesium is a mineral that plays a role in muscle function and relaxation, including the smooth muscles of the airways. Adequate magnesium intake may help reduce airway hyperresponsiveness and improve asthma symptoms.

- Include magnesium-rich foods in your diet, such as leafy greens (spinach, Swiss chard, kale), nuts (almonds, cashews), seeds (pumpkin seeds, sunflower seeds), whole grains (brown rice, quinoa, oats), legumes (beans, lentils), and dark chocolate.

5. Probiotic-Rich Foods:

- Probiotics are beneficial bacteria that support gut health and immune function. Emerging research suggests that probiotics may help reduce asthma symptoms and inflammation.

- Consume probiotic-rich foods such as yogurt (with live active cultures), kefir, fermented vegetables (sauerkraut, kimchi), kombucha, and miso soup.

6. Quercetin-Rich Foods:

- Quercetin is a flavonoid with antioxidant and anti-inflammatory properties. It may help stabilize mast cells and reduce histamine release, potentially alleviating allergic reactions and asthma symptoms.

- Enjoy quercetin-rich foods such as apples, onions, garlic, citrus fruits (especially citrus peel), berries, cherries, grapes, broccoli, leafy greens, and green tea.

Incorporating these asthma-friendly foods and nutrients into your diet can help support respiratory health, reduce inflammation, and improve asthma control. Aim for a varied and balanced diet that includes a wide range of nutrient-dense foods to optimize overall health and well-being. If you have specific dietary concerns or restrictions, consult with a registered dietitian or healthcare provider for personalized nutrition guidance tailored to your individual needs.

Tips for Meal Planning and Navigating Dietary Restrictions

Meal planning and navigating dietary restrictions can be challenging, especially for individuals with asthma who may need to be mindful of certain foods that can trigger symptoms or exacerbate inflammation. However, with careful planning and creativity, it's possible to create nutritious and satisfying meals that support respiratory health while accommodating dietary needs. Here are some tips for meal planning and navigating dietary restrictions for individuals with asthma:

1. Understand Your Dietary Restrictions:
  - Identify specific foods or ingredients that trigger asthma symptoms or exacerbate inflammation in your body. Common triggers include allergens (such as dairy, gluten, soy, eggs, shellfish), sulfites (found in processed foods and wine), and high-sodium or high-sugar foods.

- Keep a food diary to track your intake and monitor how different foods affect your asthma symptoms. This can help you pinpoint specific triggers and make informed choices when planning meals.

2. Focus on Whole, Nutrient-Dense Foods:
- Build your meals around whole, nutrient-dense foods that support respiratory health and overall well-being. Include plenty of fruits, vegetables, whole grains, lean proteins, and healthy fats in your diet.
- Choose a variety of colorful fruits and vegetables to ensure you're getting a diverse range of vitamins, minerals, and antioxidants that help reduce inflammation and support immune function.

3. Read Food Labels:
- Learn how to read food labels and ingredient lists to identify potential allergens, additives, or preservatives that may trigger asthma symptoms. Avoid packaged and processed foods with long lists of artificial ingredients and opt for whole, minimally processed foods whenever possible.

4. Experiment with Asthma-Friendly Recipes:
- Explore asthma-friendly recipes and experiment with different ingredients and flavor combinations to create meals

that suit your taste preferences and dietary needs. Look for recipes that focus on whole foods and incorporate anti-inflammatory ingredients such as fruits, vegetables, herbs, and spices.

- Get creative with substitutions for common allergens or trigger foods. For example, use dairy-free alternatives such as almond milk or coconut yogurt in place of cow's milk or yogurt, or substitute gluten-free grains like quinoa or brown rice for wheat-based grains.

5. Plan Ahead:

- Take time to plan your meals and snacks for the week ahead, considering your dietary restrictions and nutritional needs. Make a grocery list based on your meal plan and stock up on pantry staples and fresh produce.

- Preparing meals in advance can save time and reduce stress during busy weekdays. Consider batch-cooking large quantities of soups, stews, or grain-based salads that can be portioned out and enjoyed throughout the week.

6. Stay Flexible:

- Be flexible and adaptable with your meal planning, especially when dining out or attending social events. Research restaurant menus in advance, ask about ingredient substitutions or modifications, and communicate your dietary needs with the waitstaff.

- Don't be afraid to advocate for yourself and ask questions about how dishes are prepared or if certain ingredients can be omitted. Most restaurants are willing to accommodate dietary restrictions with advance notice.

7. Seek Support:

- Don't hesitate to seek support from a registered dietitian or healthcare provider who can provide personalized nutrition guidance tailored to your individual needs and dietary restrictions. They can help you develop a well-balanced meal plan that supports respiratory health while addressing any specific dietary concerns or limitations.

By following these tips for meal planning and navigating dietary restrictions, individuals with asthma can enjoy a varied and nutritious diet that supports respiratory health, reduces inflammation, and improves asthma control. With creativity, flexibility, and support from healthcare professionals, managing dietary restrictions can become an empowering part of living a healthy and fulfilling lifestyle with asthma.

CHAPTER 6: Stress Management: Coping with Emotional and Environmental Triggers

Stress can have a significant impact on asthma symptoms, exacerbating respiratory issues and triggering flare-ups. In this chapter, we'll explore the connection between stress and asthma symptoms, techniques for managing stress and anxiety to reduce asthma flare-ups, and the importance of creating a self-care routine to promote emotional well-being.

Exploring the Connection between Stress and Asthma Symptoms

The relationship between stress and asthma symptoms is complex and multifaceted. Stress can have a significant impact on the respiratory system, exacerbating asthma symptoms and triggering flare-ups. Understanding how stress affects asthma can empower individuals to better manage their condition and improve overall well-being. Here's a closer look at the connection between stress and asthma symptoms:

- **Physiological Response:**

When the body experiences stress, it activates the "fight or flight" response, also known as the stress response. This physiological reaction involves the release of stress hormones such as adrenaline and cortisol, which prepare the body to confront or flee from perceived threats.

- **Effects on the Respiratory System:**

Stress can affect the respiratory system in several ways, leading to changes in breathing patterns, lung function, and airway inflammation. During times of stress, individuals may experience rapid, shallow breathing or hyperventilation, which can trigger asthma symptoms such as wheezing, coughing, and shortness of breath.

- **Airway Constriction:**

Stress-induced changes in breathing patterns can contribute to airway constriction and bronchoconstriction, making it harder for individuals with asthma to breathe. Constricted airways are more sensitive to asthma triggers such as allergens, pollutants, and respiratory infections, increasing the risk of asthma flare-ups.

- **Inflammatory Response:**

Chronic stress has been linked to systemic inflammation, which can exacerbate airway inflammation in individuals with asthma. Inflammation plays a central role in asthma pathogenesis, contributing to airway hyperresponsiveness, mucus production, and bronchial smooth muscle contraction.

- **Psychological Factors:**

In addition to physiological effects, stress can also impact asthma symptoms through psychological mechanisms. Emotional stressors such as anxiety, depression, anger, and frustration can trigger or worsen asthma symptoms by influencing breathing patterns, immune function, and inflammatory responses.

- **Bidirectional Relationship:**

The relationship between stress and asthma is bidirectional, meaning that stress can worsen asthma symptoms, and asthma symptoms can, in turn, increase stress levels. The cycle of stress and asthma exacerbations can create a vicious cycle, with each exacerbation leading to increased stress and worsening symptoms.

- **Individual Variability:**

It's important to recognize that the impact of stress on asthma symptoms can vary widely among individuals. Some people may be more sensitive to stress-related triggers, while others may experience minimal effects. Factors such as asthma severity, coping mechanisms, social support, and overall resilience can influence how stress affects asthma control.

Understanding the connection between stress and asthma symptoms is essential for effectively managing the condition. By implementing stress management techniques, cultivating emotional resilience, and developing coping strategies, individuals with asthma can reduce the impact of stress on their respiratory health and improve overall quality of life. Additionally, integrating holistic approaches to asthma management that address both physical and psychological aspects of the condition can lead to better outcomes and enhanced well-being.

Techniques for Managing Stress and Anxiety to Reduce Asthma Flare-ups

Stress and anxiety can exacerbate asthma symptoms and trigger flare-ups. Therefore, learning effective stress management techniques is essential for individuals with asthma to reduce the impact of stress on their respiratory health and improve asthma control. Here are several techniques for managing stress and anxiety to reduce asthma flare-ups:

1. Deep Breathing Exercises:
- Deep breathing exercises, such as diaphragmatic breathing or belly breathing, can help promote relaxation and reduce stress-induced hyperventilation. Practice deep breathing by inhaling deeply through your nose, filling your abdomen with air, and then exhaling slowly through your mouth. Repeat this pattern for several minutes to calm your mind and body.

2. Mindfulness Meditation:
- Mindfulness meditation involves focusing your attention on the present moment without judgment or attachment to thoughts and emotions. Mindfulness practices can help reduce stress and anxiety by cultivating awareness, acceptance, and inner peace. Set aside time each day to practice mindfulness meditation, either through guided meditation sessions or self-directed practice.

3. Progressive Muscle Relaxation (PMR):

- Progressive muscle relaxation techniques involve systematically tensing and relaxing different muscle groups in the body to release tension and promote physical and mental relaxation. Start by tensing specific muscle groups for a few seconds, then release the tension and notice the sensation of relaxation. Work your way through the entire body, from head to toe, to achieve a state of deep relaxation.

4. Yoga and Tai Chi:

- Yoga and tai chi are gentle mind-body practices that combine physical postures, breathwork, and mindfulness to promote relaxation and reduce stress. These practices can help improve flexibility, balance, and overall well-being while calming the mind and reducing anxiety. Consider attending yoga or tai chi classes or following instructional videos online to learn the basics and incorporate these practices into your routine.

5. Cognitive Behavioral Therapy (CBT):

- Cognitive-behavioral therapy (CBT) is a type of psychotherapy that focuses on identifying and challenging negative thought patterns and developing coping skills to manage stress and anxiety. CBT techniques, such as cognitive restructuring, relaxation training, and stress management skills, can be beneficial for individuals with asthma who experience stress-related symptoms.

6. Biofeedback:

- Biofeedback is a therapeutic technique that helps individuals learn to control physiological processes such as heart rate, muscle tension, and breathing patterns through real-time feedback. Biofeedback training can teach individuals to regulate their stress response and promote relaxation, which may help reduce asthma flare-ups triggered by stress and anxiety.

7. Exercise and Physical Activity:

- Regular exercise and physical activity can help reduce stress and anxiety levels while improving overall respiratory health and asthma control. Engage in activities you enjoy, such as walking, cycling, swimming, or dancing, to release endorphins, boost mood, and alleviate symptoms of stress and anxiety.

8. Relaxation Techniques:

- Incorporate relaxation techniques into your daily routine to promote emotional well-being and reduce stress levels. These may include listening to calming music, practicing guided imagery or visualization, taking warm baths, spending time in nature, or engaging in hobbies and activities that bring you joy and relaxation.

By incorporating these stress management techniques into your daily routine, you can reduce the impact of stress and anxiety on your asthma symptoms, improve respiratory health, and enhance overall well-being. Experiment with different techniques to find what works best for you, and remember to prioritize self-care and emotional resilience as part of your asthma management plan. If you're unsure where to start or need additional support, consider seeking guidance from a healthcare provider, therapist, or stress management specialist.

Creating a Self-Care Routine to Promote Emotional Well-being

Self-care is essential for maintaining emotional well-being, reducing stress, and improving overall quality of life, especially for individuals with asthma who may experience heightened emotional and physical challenges. By prioritizing self-care and incorporating nurturing practices into your daily routine, you can better manage stress, anxiety, and asthma symptoms. Here are some tips for creating a self-care routine to promote emotional well-being:

1. Identify Your Needs:

- Take time to reflect on your emotional needs and identify activities or practices that help you feel grounded, relaxed, and rejuvenated. Consider what brings you joy, calmness, and fulfillment, and prioritize activities that nourish your mind, body, and spirit.

2. Establish Daily Rituals:

- Develop daily rituals that promote self-care and emotional well-being. Set aside dedicated time each day for activities such as mindfulness meditation, journaling, deep breathing exercises, or spending time in nature. Consistency is key to establishing healthy habits and reaping the benefits of self-care.

3. Practice Gratitude:

- Cultivate gratitude by focusing on the positive aspects of your life and expressing appreciation for the people, experiences, and blessings you're grateful for. Keep a gratitude journal and write down three things you're thankful for each day, no matter how small or ordinary they may seem.

4. Set Boundaries:

- Establish clear boundaries to protect your emotional well-being and prevent burnout. Learn to say no to commitments or obligations that drain your energy or contribute to stress. Prioritize activities and relationships that align with your values and bring you joy and fulfillment.

5. Engage in Activities You Enjoy:

- Make time for activities and hobbies that bring you pleasure and relaxation. Whether it's reading, listening to music, cooking, gardening, or engaging in creative pursuits, prioritize activities that nourish your soul and allow you to recharge and unwind.

6. Connect with Others:

- Nurture meaningful connections with friends, family members, or support groups who provide emotional support, encouragement, and companionship. Share your thoughts, feelings, and experiences with trusted individuals who understand and validate your emotions.

7. Practice Self-Compassion:

- Be kind and compassionate toward yourself, especially during challenging times. Acknowledge your strengths, accomplishments, and efforts, and treat yourself with the same kindness and understanding you would offer to a friend facing similar struggles.

8. Prioritize Sleep:

- Ensure you get an adequate amount of restorative sleep each night to support emotional well-being and overall health. Establish a relaxing bedtime routine, create a comfortable sleep environment, and prioritize sleep hygiene practices such as limiting screen time before bed and avoiding caffeine and heavy meals close to bedtime.

9. Move Your Body:

- Engage in regular physical activity to boost mood, reduce stress, and improve emotional well-being. Find activities you enjoy, such as walking, jogging, yoga, or dancing, and make movement a regular part of your self-care routine.

10. Seek Professional Support:

- Don't hesitate to seek support from a therapist, counselor, or mental health professional if you're struggling to cope with stress, anxiety, or emotional challenges. Therapy can provide a safe and supportive space to explore your feelings, learn coping skills, and develop strategies for managing stress and improving emotional resilience.

By incorporating these self-care practices into your daily routine, you can promote emotional well-being, reduce stress, and enhance overall quality of life, while also supporting asthma management and respiratory health. Remember that self-care is not selfish—it's essential for maintaining balance, resilience, and vitality in the face of life's challenges. Start small, be consistent, and prioritize self-care as an integral part of your asthma management plan.

CHAPTER 7: Support Systems: Building a Strong Asthma Support Network

Support systems play a crucial role in managing asthma effectively. This chapter explores the importance of communication with healthcare providers, family, and friends, finding support groups and online communities for individuals with asthma, and tips for advocating for yourself and others in managing asthma.

Importance of Communication with Healthcare Providers, Family, and Friends

Communication plays a vital role in managing asthma effectively and ensuring optimal health outcomes. Establishing open and honest lines of communication with healthcare providers, family members, and friends is essential for navigating the challenges associated with asthma.

Here's why communication is crucial in each of these areas:

- **Healthcare Providers:**

- Effective communication with healthcare providers is essential for accurate diagnosis, personalized treatment plans, and ongoing management of asthma symptoms. Your healthcare team, which may include primary care physicians, pulmonologists, allergists, and asthma educators, relies on your input to make informed decisions about your care.

- By openly discussing your symptoms, triggers, medication use, and treatment preferences with your healthcare providers, you can work together to develop a comprehensive asthma management plan tailored to your specific needs. Regular check-ups and follow-up appointments provide opportunities to assess your asthma control, adjust treatment as needed, and address any concerns or questions you may have.

- Don't hesitate to ask questions or seek clarification about your asthma diagnosis, treatment options, medication instructions, and self-management strategies. Your healthcare providers are there to support you and provide guidance every step of the way.

- **Family:**

- Family members play a crucial role in supporting individuals with asthma and helping them manage their condition effectively. Open communication with family members about your asthma diagnosis, symptoms, triggers, and treatment plan can foster understanding, empathy, and cooperation within the household.

- Educate family members about asthma, including common symptoms, triggers, and emergency response protocols. Encourage them to participate in asthma education programs or attend appointments with you to learn more about how they can support your asthma management efforts.

- Collaborate with family members to create an asthma-friendly environment at home by minimizing exposure to allergens, pollutants, and irritants that may trigger asthma symptoms. Work together to develop an asthma action plan that outlines steps to take in case of an asthma exacerbation or emergency.

- **Friends:**

- Friends can also provide valuable support and encouragement for individuals living with asthma. Be open and honest with your friends about your asthma diagnosis and how it affects your daily life, activities, and social interactions.

- Communicate your needs and preferences to friends when planning social outings or activities. Let them know if you have any specific triggers or concerns related to asthma, such as exposure to smoke, pet dander, or strong odors.

- Consider enlisting the support of close friends who can help you stay accountable with medication adherence, remind you to carry your rescue inhaler, or provide assistance during asthma flare-ups or emergencies.

Overall, effective communication with healthcare providers, family, and friends fosters a supportive network that empowers individuals with asthma to manage their condition effectively, minimize triggers, and lead healthy, fulfilling lives. Don't hesitate to reach out for support or guidance whenever you need it, and remember that you're not alone in your asthma journey.

Finding Support Groups and Online Communities for Individuals with Asthma

Navigating life with asthma can be challenging, but finding support from others who understand your experiences can make a significant difference. Support groups and online communities provide valuable opportunities for individuals with asthma to connect with peers, share insights, and access resources and information. Here's how to find and benefit from these supportive networks:

1. Local Support Groups:

- Start by checking with local hospitals, clinics, or community centers to see if there are any asthma support groups or programs available in your area. These groups may offer in-person meetings, educational workshops, and social events where you can connect with others who have asthma.

- Local support groups provide a sense of community and camaraderie, allowing you to share experiences, exchange tips for managing asthma, and learn from each other's successes and challenges. Meeting face-to-face with fellow asthma sufferers can be especially valuable for building relationships and finding encouragement.

2. National Organizations:

- Explore national organizations dedicated to asthma advocacy and support, such as the American Lung Association (ALA), Asthma and Allergy Foundation of America (AAFA), and Allergy & Asthma Network. These organizations often offer resources, educational materials, and online support communities for individuals with asthma and their families.

- Visit the websites of these organizations to access information about asthma management, treatment options, asthma action plans, and coping strategies. Many organizations also host webinars, forums, and virtual support groups where you can connect with others from the comfort of your home.

3. Online Communities:

- Join online communities and forums specifically tailored to individuals with asthma. Websites such as Inspire, Asthma UK's HealthUnlocked, and Reddit's Asthma subreddit provide platforms for sharing experiences, asking questions, and seeking advice from a global community of asthma sufferers.

- Participate in discussions, share your own insights and tips for managing asthma, and learn from the experiences of others. Online communities offer a supportive space where you can connect with people who understand the daily challenges of living with asthma and offer empathy and encouragement.

4. Social Media Groups:

- Search for asthma-related groups and pages on social media platforms such as Facebook, Twitter, and Instagram. These groups may be public or private and can vary in focus, from general asthma support to specific topics such as asthma and exercise, asthma in children, or severe asthma management.

- Follow reputable organizations, healthcare professionals, and advocacy groups specializing in asthma on social media to stay informed about the latest research, news, and events related to asthma care and advocacy.

5. Attend Asthma Events and Workshops:

- Keep an eye out for asthma-related events, conferences, and workshops in your area or online. These events may feature guest speakers, expert panels, and networking opportunities where you can connect with other individuals with asthma, caregivers, and healthcare professionals.
- Check the websites of local hospitals, medical centers, universities, and asthma advocacy organizations for information about upcoming events and how to register or participate.

By actively engaging with support groups and online communities for individuals with asthma, you can gain valuable insights, practical tips, and emotional support to help you better manage your condition and live well with asthma. Whether you're seeking advice, sharing your experiences, or simply connecting with others who understand what you're going through, these supportive networks can be invaluable resources on your asthma journey.

Tips for Advocating for Yourself and Others in Managing Asthma

Advocacy plays a crucial role in ensuring that individuals with asthma receive the support, resources, and care they need to effectively manage their condition and lead healthy lives. Whether advocating for yourself or supporting others with asthma, here are some tips for being an effective advocate:

1. Educate Yourself:
  - Take the time to educate yourself about asthma, including its causes, symptoms, triggers, treatment options, and self-management strategies. Knowledge is power, and being well-informed empowers you to make informed decisions about your care and advocate effectively for your needs.

2. Know Your Rights:
  - Familiarize yourself with your rights as a person with asthma, including protections under the Americans with Disabilities Act (ADA) and other relevant legislation. Understand your entitlements to reasonable

accommodations, workplace protections, and access to healthcare services and resources.

3. Communicate Effectively:

- Practice clear and assertive communication when discussing your asthma needs with healthcare providers, employers, educators, and others. Clearly articulate your symptoms, triggers, treatment preferences, and any concerns or questions you may have.

- Be proactive in seeking information, asking questions, and advocating for yourself during medical appointments, meetings, and interactions with healthcare professionals.

4. Keep Records:

- Maintain organized records of your asthma management, including medication schedules, symptom diaries, asthma action plans, and medical history. Documenting your asthma-related experiences can help track trends, identify triggers, and provide valuable information for healthcare providers.

- Keep copies of relevant medical reports, test results, prescriptions, and correspondence with healthcare providers for reference and documentation purposes.

5. Develop an Asthma Action Plan:

- Work with your healthcare provider to develop a personalized asthma action plan that outlines steps to take for asthma prevention, symptom management, and emergency response. Share your asthma action plan with family members, caregivers, teachers, and others who may need to assist you during an asthma exacerbation.

- Advocate for the implementation of asthma-friendly policies and practices in schools, workplaces, and other community settings to ensure access to asthma medications, accommodations for asthma triggers, and emergency preparedness.

6. Seek Support:

- Don't hesitate to seek support from healthcare professionals, advocacy organizations, support groups, and online communities specializing in asthma. These resources can provide guidance, information, and emotional support to help you navigate the challenges of living with asthma and advocating for your needs.

- Connect with other individuals with asthma, caregivers, and advocates to share experiences, exchange insights, and collaborate on advocacy initiatives aimed at improving asthma awareness, education, and care.

7. Raise Awareness:

- Take advantage of opportunities to raise awareness about asthma and advocate for greater understanding, acceptance, and support for individuals with asthma. Share your story, participate in asthma awareness campaigns, and engage in advocacy efforts to promote asthma research, funding, and policy initiatives.

- Use social media, community events, and other platforms to amplify your voice, advocate for positive change, and challenge stigma and misconceptions surrounding asthma.

8. Be Persistent:

- Advocacy is often a long-term process that requires persistence, patience, and resilience. Don't be discouraged by setbacks or challenges along the way. Stay focused on your goals, continue advocating for yourself and others, and celebrate small victories and successes along the journey.

By advocating for yourself and others in managing asthma, you can help improve awareness, access to care, and quality of life for individuals living with this chronic condition. Remember that your voice matters, and together, we can work toward a future where everyone with asthma receives the support and resources they need to thrive.

CHAPTER 8: Overcoming Obstacles: Thriving with Asthma Despite Challenges

Living with asthma presents unique challenges, but with determination, resilience, and support, individuals can overcome obstacles and thrive despite their condition. This chapter explores common misconceptions and stigma surrounding asthma, strategies for overcoming barriers to asthma management, and inspiring stories of individuals who have overcome obstacles to live fulfilling lives with asthma.

Addressing Common Misconceptions and Stigma Surrounding Asthma

Asthma is a chronic respiratory condition that affects millions of people worldwide, yet it is often misunderstood and surrounded by stigma and misconceptions. Addressing these misconceptions and challenging the stigma surrounding asthma is essential for promoting understanding, empathy, and support for individuals living with the condition. Here are some common misconceptions about asthma and strategies for addressing them:

1. Asthma is Just a Minor Condition:

- Misconception: Some people believe that asthma is a minor inconvenience or simply a condition that causes occasional wheezing or shortness of breath.

- Reality: Asthma is a chronic inflammatory condition of the airways that can vary widely in severity and impact. For many individuals, asthma can be a serious and potentially life-threatening condition that requires ongoing management and treatment.

2. Asthma Only Affects Children:

- Misconception: There is a common belief that asthma is primarily a childhood condition that children outgrow as they get older.

- Reality: While asthma often begins in childhood, it can affect people of all ages, from infants to older adults. Many individuals continue to experience asthma symptoms and require treatment into adulthood, and some may develop asthma for the first time later in life.

3. Asthma Can Be Cured Through Lifestyle Changes:

- Misconception: Some people believe that asthma can be cured or effectively managed through lifestyle changes alone, such as avoiding triggers or adopting a healthy diet and exercise routine.

- Reality: While lifestyle modifications can help improve asthma control and reduce symptoms, asthma is a chronic condition that typically requires ongoing medical treatment, including medication and regular monitoring by healthcare providers.

4. Asthma Is Contagious:

- Misconception: There is a misconception that asthma is contagious and can be spread from person to person through close contact or sharing items such as food, drinks, or personal belongings.

- Reality: Asthma is not contagious and cannot be transmitted from one person to another. Asthma is believed to result from a combination of genetic, environmental, and immune system factors, and it is not caused by exposure to individuals with the condition.

5. People with Asthma Should Avoid Physical Activity:

- Misconception: Some people believe that individuals with asthma should avoid physical activity or exercise because it can trigger asthma symptoms or exacerbate breathing difficulties.

- Reality: Regular physical activity is important for overall health and well-being, including for individuals with asthma. With proper management and appropriate precautions, most people with asthma can safely participate in physical activity and enjoy the benefits of exercise.

Strategies for Addressing Misconceptions and Stigma:

1. Education and Awareness:

- Provide accurate information and education about asthma to dispel myths and misconceptions. Use trusted sources such as healthcare professionals, reputable medical organizations, and peer-reviewed literature to share facts and evidence-based information about asthma.

2. Open Dialogue and Communication:

- Encourage open dialogue and communication about asthma in families, schools, workplaces, and communities. Foster discussions that promote understanding, empathy, and support for individuals living with asthma and their families.

3. Storytelling and Personal Narratives:

- Share personal stories and experiences of individuals living with asthma to humanize the condition and raise awareness about its impact on daily life. Personal narratives can help challenge stereotypes, combat stigma, and foster empathy and understanding.

4. Advocacy and Policy Change:

- Advocate for policies and initiatives that promote asthma awareness, education, and support. Support efforts to improve access to healthcare services, medications, and resources for individuals with asthma, particularly in underserved communities.

5. Community Engagement and Support:

- Engage with community organizations, advocacy groups, and online communities dedicated to asthma awareness and support. Participate in events, campaigns, and initiatives that raise awareness about asthma and advocate for positive change.

By addressing common misconceptions and challenging the stigma surrounding asthma, we can create a more inclusive and supportive environment for individuals living with the condition. Through education, advocacy, and community engagement, we can promote understanding, empathy, and acceptance for all those affected by asthma.

Strategies for Overcoming Barriers to Asthma Management

Living with asthma requires access to proper medical care, medications, and resources for effective management. However, financial constraints, lack of access to healthcare, and other barriers can hinder individuals' ability to receive the care they need. Here are strategies to overcome these barriers and ensure adequate asthma management:

1. Seek Affordable Healthcare Options:

- Explore affordable healthcare options available in your area, such as community health centers, clinics, and free or low-cost healthcare services. These facilities often offer sliding-scale fees or discounted rates based on income and can provide essential asthma care, including diagnosis, treatment, and management.

2. Utilize Patient Assistance Programs:

- Many pharmaceutical companies offer patient assistance programs that provide free or discounted medications to individuals who cannot afford them. These programs may cover asthma medications, including inhalers, controller medications, and rescue medications. Check with your healthcare provider or the medication manufacturer for information on available assistance programs.

3. Access Public Health Programs:

- Take advantage of public health programs and initiatives that support individuals with asthma, such as state-based asthma programs, asthma education programs, and home visitation services. These programs may offer resources, education, and support to help manage asthma effectively and reduce barriers to care.

4. Explore Telehealth Services:

- Telehealth services, including virtual doctor visits and telemedicine consultations, can provide convenient and accessible healthcare options for individuals with asthma, particularly those facing geographic or transportation barriers. Many healthcare providers offer telehealth appointments for routine asthma care, medication management, and follow-up visits.

5. Advocate for Expanded Healthcare Access:

- Advocate for policies and initiatives that expand access to healthcare services, medications, and resources for individuals with asthma. Support efforts to improve healthcare infrastructure, increase funding for asthma programs, and expand insurance coverage to ensure equitable access to care for all individuals, regardless of socioeconomic status.

6. Educate Yourself and Empower Others:

- Take an active role in educating yourself about asthma management, treatment options, and self-care strategies. Empower yourself with knowledge and resources to effectively manage your asthma and advocate for your needs within the healthcare system.

- Share information and resources with others in your community who may be facing similar barriers to asthma management. Offer support, guidance, and encouragement to empower individuals to take control of their asthma and access the care they need.

7. Access Community Resources and Support:

- Connect with community organizations, advocacy groups, and support networks dedicated to asthma awareness and support. These organizations may offer resources, educational materials, support groups, and financial assistance programs to help individuals overcome barriers to asthma management.

- Collaborate with community partners, healthcare providers, and local stakeholders to develop and implement initiatives that address systemic barriers to asthma care, such as lack of access to healthcare, limited transportation options, or language barriers.

By implementing these strategies and advocating for expanded access to healthcare, medications, and resources, individuals with asthma can overcome barriers to care and effectively manage their condition. Together, we can work to ensure that all individuals have the support they need to live healthy, fulfilling lives with asthma.

Inspiring Stories of Individuals Overcoming Obstacles to Live Fulfilling Lives with Asthma

Despite the challenges presented by asthma, many individuals have demonstrated remarkable resilience, determination, and courage in overcoming obstacles to lead fulfilling lives. Here are a few inspiring stories of individuals who have navigated the ups and downs of living with asthma and achieved their goals:

- **Michael Phelps:**
  - Michael Phelps, the most decorated Olympian of all time, has asthma. Despite his condition, he pursued his passion

for swimming and became a record-breaking athlete, winning 28 Olympic medals, including 23 gold medals. Phelps has spoken openly about his asthma diagnosis and how he managed his condition while training and competing at the highest level of professional sports.

- **Kristin Chenoweth:**

  - Kristin Chenoweth, an award-winning actress and singer, has asthma and allergies. Despite facing challenges related to her health, she has achieved success on Broadway, in film, and on television. Chenoweth has been an advocate for asthma awareness and has spoken publicly about her experiences managing her condition while pursuing her career in the entertainment industry.

- **Jerome Bettis:**

  - Jerome Bettis, a former professional football player and Super Bowl champion, was diagnosed with asthma as a child. Despite facing asthma-related challenges, he excelled in football and became one of the most celebrated running backs in NFL history. Bettis has been an advocate for asthma awareness and has shared his story to inspire others living with the condition.

- **Kathy Bates:**

- Kathy Bates, an Academy Award-winning actress, was diagnosed with asthma later in life. Despite her diagnosis, she has continued to pursue her passion for acting and has achieved success in film, television, and theater. Bates has been vocal about her experiences managing asthma and has encouraged others to seek proper diagnosis and treatment.

- **Vanessa Williams:**

- Vanessa Williams, a singer, actress, and former Miss America, was diagnosed with asthma as a child. Despite facing challenges related to her health, she has enjoyed a successful career in the entertainment industry, with hit songs, acclaimed performances, and numerous accolades. Williams has spoken openly about her asthma diagnosis and how she manages her condition while balancing her career and personal life.

These are just a few examples of individuals who have overcome obstacles to live fulfilling lives with asthma. Their stories serve as powerful reminders that asthma does not have to define or limit one's potential. With proper management, support, and determination, individuals with asthma can pursue their passions, achieve their goals, and thrive in all aspects of life. These inspiring individuals serve as role models for others living with asthma, demonstrating that with resilience and perseverance, anything is possible.

CHAPTER 10: Looking to the Future: Empowering Yourself for Long-Term Asthma Wellness

As you embark on your journey towards long-term asthma wellness, it's important to reflect on the key strategies for managing asthma effectively, continue prioritizing self-care and advocacy, and embrace the possibilities of living beyond the limits of asthma. In this final chapter, we recap essential strategies, offer encouragement for ongoing self-care and advocacy, and share final thoughts on embracing life with asthma:

Recap of Key Strategies for Managing Asthma Effectively:

1. Medication Management: Work closely with your healthcare team to develop a personalized asthma treatment plan, including medications, inhalers, and other therapies. Adhere to your prescribed medication regimen and attend regular check-ups to monitor your asthma control.

2. Lifestyle Modifications: Identify and minimize asthma triggers in your environment, create an asthma action plan for daily management, and incorporate asthma-friendly habits into your daily routine. Prioritize self-care practices such as stress management, exercise, nutrition, and sleep hygiene.

3. Support Systems: Build a strong support network of healthcare providers, family, friends, and peer support groups. Advocate for yourself and others in managing asthma, seek out community resources and support, and raise awareness about asthma to combat stigma and misconceptions.

Encouragement for Continued Self-Care and Advocacy:

1. Stay Informed: Continue educating yourself about asthma management, treatment advances, and self-care strategies. Stay up-to-date on the latest research, guidelines, and resources available for individuals with asthma.

2. Prioritize Self-Care: Keep prioritizing self-care practices that promote physical, emotional, and mental well-being.

Take time for relaxation, exercise, hobbies, and activities that bring you joy and fulfillment.

3. Advocate for Change: Keep advocating for policies and initiatives that support individuals with asthma, improve access to healthcare services, and promote asthma awareness and education. Your voice matters, and your advocacy efforts can make a difference in the lives of others living with asthma.

Final Thoughts on Living Beyond the Limits of Asthma:

Living with asthma is a journey filled with challenges, but it's also an opportunity to cultivate resilience, strength, and empowerment. Despite the obstacles you may face, remember that you are not defined by your asthma. You are capable of achieving your goals, pursuing your passions, and living a fulfilling life beyond the limits of asthma.

Embrace each day as an opportunity to thrive, to connect with others, and to make a positive impact in the world. Celebrate your victories, no matter how small, and lean on your support network during times of challenge. With perseverance, determination, and the support of others, you can overcome obstacles, manage asthma effectively, and live life to the fullest.

As you look to the future, remember that you are not alone on this journey. Your healthcare team, your loved ones, and your community are here to support you every step of the way. Keep empowering yourself, advocating for your needs, and embracing the possibilities of living beyond the limits of asthma. Your story is unique, valuable, and full of potential. Seize each moment, and continue writing your own inspiring chapter in the book of asthma wellness.